Contents

What Is a Tagine?

A tagine, sometimes spelled "tajine," is a traditional Moroccan cooking vessel made of ceramic or unglazed clay with a round base and low sides. A cone-shaped cover sits on the base during cooking. The conical lid traps steam during cooking and returns the liquid to the clay pot, resulting in a moist dish with concentrated flavors.

Tagine is also the name for a Maghrebi, or North African, dish cooked in the tagine pot. Tagine is closely associated with Moroccan cuisine, where slow-cooked savory stews made with meat, poultry, or fish, are cooked with vegetables, aromatic spices, dried fruit, and nuts.

The origin of Tagine

The word Tajine or Moroccan Tagine is a distinctive earthenware dish with two parts; a pose unit which is flat and circular with low sides and a large cone, or dome-shaped covers that rests inside the base during cooking. In that clay dish with a cone shaped top it is cooked and served. The word Tajine or Tagine can refer to both: food, prepared in that dish or to the dish.

The history of "Moroccan tajine" is debated. It has been suggested that tajine was first introduced to Morocco in the 12th century by the Phoenicians, who visited the area in that time. While another theory attributes it to Tonac civilization that was in Mexico between the 800 and 600 B.C.This theory based its assumption on the statuette of "EL Tagine" the god of rain of that civilization. However, the most plausible evidence attributed it to North Africa and its first settler's -Berber.

Whatever your belief as to the origin of the couscous and Tajine, the most notable Moroccan dishes, they by any name and origin taste great.

Moroccan Tajine and couscous are two faces to the same coin; it is the delicacy of Moroccan cuisine. They are two national dishes that take great advantages from the strong Andalusian, Jewish's influence and from the natural bounty.

More than any other food, couscous, the most popular dish around the world, is cooked in restaurants as in houses with pumped semolina grain and different vegetables and it is served on a clay platter called, Gues 'in a heaped pyramid style with a hollow on top which is filled with stew and embellished by multi-colored vegetables, pleasing the eye before pleasing the stomach; why not watering the mouth, and it is that baby that has come to existence after a long partition of ten centuries from its Hispano, Jewish and Muslim mother.

Tajine is a no less important dish than the couscous. Moroccans believe that no other country's dish has reached the exalted height of their Moroccan Tajine. Aromatic; stimulating fragrant, zesty, spicy or sweet, Moroccan delectable vegetables Tajine is constantly delicious and inviting for its savoring ingredients, which may include, depending on the genre of the Tajine, lamb or poultry stew, almond, hard boiled eggs, burns, lemons, potatoes, carrots, onions, tomatoes and spices including saffron, cumin, coriander, ginger, red pepper...and cinnamon. These components with others, produce an enticing aroma as they are cooked in a clay plat with a cone-shaped top.

Thanks to its delicate flavor its exceptional nutritive virtues and the conviviality it creates, Moroccan Tajine celebrates its leadership in the world of gastronomy. Undoubtedly, the one who has just eaten a Moroccan couscous or Tajine, will yearn to sample once again other distinctive, flavoring and simmering dishes somewhere in a wide range of Moroccan restaurants and will ask for recipes to take them with him.

How to Use a Tagine

Follow this step-by-step guide to using a tagine.

1. Season the tagine. A tagine should be seasoned before using to strengthen and seal it, and, if it is unglazed, to remove the taste of raw clay. To season, soak the lid and base in water for 2 hours. Dry the tagine and brush the interior and exterior of the lid and base with olive oil. Place the cookware in a cold oven and set the oven to 300°F. Bake for two hours, then turn off the oven and let tagine completely cool inside. Wash the tagine and brush once more with olive oil before using it.

2. Make the base layer. The first step of cooking tagine is to place a layer of vegetables across the base of the pot, creating a cushion for the remaining ingredients. A bed of chopped onions, celery, or carrots will keep the meat from sticking to the bottom and burning during

cooking. Chopped or whole garlic cloves can be added to the base for flavor.

3. Add olive oil. Adding enough olive oil is important to make a rich sauce in tagine, most recipes recommend at least ¼ cup. You can find our complete guide to olive oil here.

4. Add meat, poultry, or fish. In the center, add meat, poultry, or fish. Arrange in a mound in the center, leaving enough room to add additional vegetables around the edges. Arrange vegetables around the meat.

5. Season with spices. Sprinkle spices generously over the meat and vegetables to make a rich, flavorful sauce. Spices that work well in tagine recipes are: cardamom, clove, cinnamon, ground coriander, cumin, paprika,

mace, nutmeg, peppercorn, ground ginger, and ground turmeric.

6. Garnish the dish. Presentation is an important part of making tagine. You can add color with strips of bell peppers, olives, or preserved lemon. Add tied bundles of fresh herbs like parsley, oregano, or cilantro.

7. Add enough water or broth. Adding liquid such as water or chicken broth to the tagine keeps food moist while cooking. Pour water or chicken stock carefully into the side of the tagine, around 1 ½ cups for a small tagine, and 2 ½ cups for a large tagine. Adjust as needed according to the recipe.

8. Cook the tagine. Avoid high heat to keep the tagine from cracking. Place it above the heat

source, not directly on it (a diffuser is needed for electric stovetops). Place over low to medium-low heat until it reaches a slow simmer. The cooking time for recipes can vary with fish and chicken being shorter, and beef and lamb taking longer.

9. Check the liquid. After 2 hours, check the level of the cooking liquid. If the liquid has already thickened, add another ¼ cup of liquid.

10. Serving the tagine. Tagines double as a beautiful serving dish. Make sure to allow the tagine to cool down for 15 minutes before serving. Traditionally, tagine is served as a dish to share communally, using Moroccan bread to scoop and up the meat, vegetables, and sauce. Tagine is also delicious served over couscous.

What Do You Need to Make the Perfect Tagine?

The Cooking Vessel

The word tagine is not only the name of the stew but is also the name of the pot in which it is prepared (perhaps a "which came first, the chicken or the egg" scenario). A Moroccan tagine consists of a shallow glazed earthenware bowl to hold all of the ingredients. But instead of a typical lid, a cone-shaped cover is placed on top.

If it's within your budget to purchase one, you can certainly find one online. (Go to the world-famous online store that sells everything on the planet). Otherwise, you can use a Dutch oven or a heavy skillet with a tight-fitting lid.

If you decide to purchase an authentic clay tagine, I would recommend that you opt for a glazed pot. Unglazed pots have a rustic beauty, but require more preparation and seasoning to maintain.

Preserved Lemon

Many tagine recipes will ask you to add preserved lemon to the dish. If you happen to live in a large metropolitan area you might be able to find these in the gourmet section of your grocery store. But, if you can't find them on your local store shelf, you can make your own.

Ingredients

- 5 organic lemons

- 1/4 cup Kosher salt
- Juice of 6 to 8 additional lemons

Instructions

1. Quarter the lemons almost all the way through from tip to tip—they should still be attached at one end. Rub salt inside each quartered lemon.

2. Pack the lemons in a sterilized quart jar. Add any salt that remains and enough lemon juice to cover.

3. Seal the jar and allow it to stand at room temperature in a dark, dry, and cool place for 14 days, inverting the jar every day. After 14 days store the jar in the refrigerator.

4. Rinse the lemons before using (use the rind only).

Ras el Hanout

The name means "head of the shop," the best spices one has to offer. Ras el hanout (pronounced "ross el hanOOT") is a spunky, savory blend that varies from region to region, house to house, and even cook to cook. The primary ingredients are coriander, cinnamon, cardamom, and peppercorn. Here is a recipe that uses nine seasonings you probably already have in your pantry. Simply blend them all together and store in a tightly lidded jar in a cool, dry place.

Ingredients

- 1 teaspoon ground cumin

- 1 teaspoon ground ginger
- 1 teaspoon table salt
- 3/4 teaspoon freshly ground black pepper
- 1/2 teaspoon ground cinnamon
- 1/2 teaspoon ground coriander seeds
- 1/2 teaspoon cayenne
- 1/2 teaspoon ground allspice
- 1/4 teaspoon ground cloves

Couscous

Couscous is made of wheat grain. For those who are sensitive to gluten, brown rice would be a perfectly great substitute.

Recipe Ideas for Your Moroccan Tagine

Now that you've mastered how to use your tagine, see below for some creative recipe ideas using your tagine.

- Moroccan lamb tagine. Tender seasoned lamb stew meat with chickpeas, dates, oranges, and almonds is a classic sweet and savory Moroccan dish. Serve over couscous to soak up its delicious sauce.

- Moroccan chicken with preserved lemons and olives. A fragrant chicken stew with spiced bone-in chicken thighs or chicken breasts cooked with tangy preserved lemons, sauteed onions, and savory green olives. Finish with sprigs of fresh cilantro.

- Moroccan chicken and apricot. The secret to this dish is using the North African spice blend, Ras El Hanout, made with cardamom, clove, ground cinnamon, coriander, ground cumin, paprika, mace, nutmeg, peppercorn, and turmeric. The spice blend adds a bold flavor to the chicken and makes a rich sauce. Dried apricots, tomatoes, and honey are added to the dish for a combination of savory and sweet.

- Kefta Mkaouara (Moroccan meatballs). A Moroccan meatball dish in a zesty tomato sauce. Eggs are often added to the dish at the end of cooking, resulting in poached eggs perfect for dipping with crusty Moroccan bread.

- Mqualli (Fish tagine). A classic fish dish with potatoes, tomatoes, and bell peppers. Any firm fish can be used such as swordfish, sea bass, or dorado. The sauce base is typically made with ginger, saffron, and extra virgin olive oil.

- Moroccan vegetable tagine. A vegetarian-friendly tagine made with chickpeas, carrots, russet potatoes, and sweet potatoes. Seasoned with harissa paste and a touch of sweetness from honey and golden raisins.

- Shakshuka. Shakshuka is a simple and delicious dish of eggs that are poached in a spiced tomato sauce that is cooked with onions, chili peppers and garnished with herbs. Shakshuka is traditionally cooked in a tagine, but it can also be made in a cast-iron pan or skillet.

- Apricot Chicken Tagine Fresh, healthy ingredients are the cornerstone of tagine cooking, and this apricot chicken stew is a perfect introduction to the concept of using a tagine. A savory combination of herbs and spices is rubbed onto the skin of chicken thighs (or drumsticks). Dark meat is really the better choice for this dish—chicken breasts would turn dry and chalky in the long simmer; chicken hindquarters emerge succulent, moist, and fall-off-the-bone tender. Tomato and lemon provide a tart, savory counter to the sweet note of dried fruits and honey.

• Lemon Olive Chicken (Djej M'Chernel) Poultry is the foundation for this savory lemon olive chicken, but it's the tangy lemon and briny olives that are the stars of the show. Green olives are picked at the start of the harvest season and are typically firmer than their black (ripe) counterparts. If you are fortunate to have a deli nearby that sells olives, look for the picholine, torpedo-shaped olives from France, that are tart and anise-y. If you cannot find those, the Manzanilla, a brine-cured crisp olive from Spain would be a good substitute.

- Eggplant and Pumpkin Tagine Do not skimp on the time to low-and-slow caramelize the onions for this eggplant pumpkin tagine. When treated with patience, onions transform from hot and biting to beautifully sweet and soft; they almost melt. With turmeric and ginger, they create a rich and comforting sauce for the creamy vegetables. Serve this over a steaming mound of couscous.

• Fish Tagine With Preserved Lemon Cooking fish in a tagine is a guarantee that the fish will always be cooked perfectly—moist, flavorful, and flaky. This recipe from the May 2006 issue of Cooking Light magazine suggests mahimahi. Halibut, sea bass, or tilapia would make excellent substitutions of mahimahi isn't available.

• Moroccan Beef Tagine We included this recipe for Moroccan beef tagine because sometimes you want a dish with the amazing flavors of tagine without the lengthy cooking time. Instead of braising cubes of beef, use lean ground beef; it's economical and has all the beefy savory flavor of stew meat without the hassle. However, don't assume that this tagine is boring—there are plenty of earthy spices, a pinch of cayenne for heat, tomato for added umami flavor, and just the right balance of sweet and tangy with apricots, raisins, olives, and preserved lemon.

- Moroccan Lamb Tagine This lamb tagine is a beautiful contrast of tastes and textures. There's a sweet edge from the dates and honey and a bit of sour from lemon juice. The softness of the lamb, cooked to perfection, is juxtaposed with the deliciously crunchy almonds. And then, a kick of hot and earthy spices as well.

- Vegetable Tagine With Almond and Chickpea Couscous This final recipe is one more gift to my vegetarian friends (and daughter) who adore the sweet/savory blend of fruit and spice that is the tagine but don't want the meat. This vegetable tagine, rich and savory with ground spices and harissa paste, sweet with honey and apricot, and scented with fresh mint, gets a protein boost with the addition of chickpeas (garbanzo beans) to the couscous accompaniment.

TAGINE RECIPES

The following recipes are tagine-friendly while also being a treat to the taste buds. Try some of these tagine diet recipes today.

Moroccan Lamb or Beef Tagine With Prunes

Prepartion time

1 hour 25 minutes

Ingredients

- 2 pounds tender beef or lamb, cut into 3-inch pieces
- 2 medium onions, grated or very finely chopped
- 3 cloves garlic, finely chopped or pressed
- 3/4 teaspoon salt
- 1 teaspoon ground black pepper
- 1 teaspoon ground ginger
- 1/2 teaspoon saffron threads, crumbled
- 1/2 teaspoon turmeric
- 1 to 2 (3- to 4-inch) pieces cinnamon stick
- 1/4 cup olive oil
- 1/4 cup butter, softened
- 2 1/2 cups water

- Handful of cilantro sprigs, tied together
- 1/2 pound prunes
- 1 tablespoon honey
- 2 tablespoons sugar
- 1 1/2 teaspoons ground cinnamon
- Optional: 1 tablespoon toasted sesame seeds
- Optional: Handful of fried almonds

Instructions

Cook the Meat

1. Gather the ingredients.

2. Pressure Cooker Moroccan Lamb or Beef Tagine With Prunes ingredients

3. In a bowl, mix the meat with the onions, garlic, and spices.

4. Heat the oil and butter in a skillet over medium heat and brown the meat for a few minutes until a crust forms.

5. Place the meat mixture in the pressure cooker and add 2 1/2 cups of water and the cilantro. Over high heat, bring the meat and liquids to a simmer.

6. Cover tightly and continue heating until pressure is achieved. Reduce the heat to medium, and cook with pressure for 45 to 50 minutes.

7. About halfway through cooking, remove 1/2 cup of the liquid and reserve.

Cook the Prunes

1. While the meat is cooking, put the prunes in a small pot and cover with water. Simmer over medium heat, partially covered, until the prunes are tender enough to easily pinch off the pit or pinch in half. (The amount of time this takes can vary greatly depending on the prunes, but the average is 15 to 30 minutes.)

2. Drain the prunes, then add the 1/2 cup of the reserved liquid from the meat.

3. Stir in the honey, sugar, and ground cinnamon, and simmer the prunes for another 5 to 10 minutes, or until they are sitting in a thick syrup.

To Serve

1. Arrange the meat on a large serving platter and spoon the prunes and syrup on top.

2. If desired, garnish with sesame seeds and/or fried almonds. Moroccan tradition is to gather around the table and eat from this communal plate, using Moroccan bread to scoop up the meat and sauce.

Moroccan Chicken Tagine

Prepartion time

3 hours 15 minutes

Ingredients

- 1 to 2 preserved lemons, quartered and seeds removed
- 1 whole chicken, cut into pieces, skin removed, back discarded or reserved for another use
- 2 large white or yellow onions, finely chopped
- 2 to 3 cloves garlic, minced
- 1 small handful fresh cilantro, chopped
- 1 small handful fresh parsley, chopped
- 2 teaspoons powdered ginger
- 1 teaspoon black pepper
- 1 teaspoon turmeric (or 1/4 teaspoon Moroccan yellow colorant)
- 1/2 teaspoon salt, or to taste

- 1/4 teaspoon saffron threads, crumbled, optional
- 1 teaspoon smen, optional
- 1/4 to 1/2 teaspoon ras el hanout, optional
- 1/3 cup olive oil
- 2 handfuls pitted olives (green or red, or mixed)
- 1/4 cup water, approximately, if using a tagine

Instructions

Marinate the Chicken

1. Gather the ingredients.

2. Remove the flesh from the preserved lemons and chop the flesh finely. Reserve rind for cooking.

3. Remove the flesh from the preserved lemons and chop the flesh finely

4. Add the lemon flesh to a bowl along with the chicken, onion, garlic, cilantro, parsley, ginger, pepper, turmeric, and salt. If using, add the saffron, ras el hanout, and smen. Mix well.

5. If time allows, let the chicken marinate in the refrigerator for several hours or overnight. Cook in either a tagine or in the oven. (See below for more information on both methods.)

Cooking in a Tagine

1. Add enough of the olive oil to the tagine to coat the bottom.

2. Arrange the marinated chicken in the tagine, flesh-side down, and distribute the onions all around.

3. Add the olives and reserved rind of the preserved lemons, and drizzle the remaining olive oil over the chicken.

4. Add the water to the tagine, cover, and place on a heat diffuser over medium-low heat. Give the tagine time to reach a simmer without peaking. If you don't hear the tagine simmering within 20 minutes, slightly increase the heat, and then use the lowest heat setting required for maintaining a gentle—not rapid—simmer.

5. Allow the chicken to cook undisturbed for 80 to 90 minutes, and then turn the chicken over so it's flesh-side up. Cover the tagine again, and allow the chicken to finish cooking until very tender (about 45 minutes to 1 hour).

6. Turn off the heat, and let the tagine cool for about 10 to 15 minutes before serving. Enjoy.

Cooking in the Oven

1. Preheat oven to 425 F/220 C. Add enough of the olive oil to a large baking dish so it coats the bottom.

2. Add enough of the olive oil to a large baking dish so it coats the bottom

3. Add the sliced onions and garlic from the marinade.

4. Then place the marinated chicken on top.

5. Add the olives and reserved rind of the preserved lemons on top and drizzle the chicken with the remaining olive oil.

6. Bake the chicken uncovered for 45 minutes to 1 hour, or until the chicken is light golden brown, basting occasionally.

7. Reduce the heat to 350 F/180 C and continue baking for another 20 to 30 minutes or longer. The chicken should be deeply browned and the juices should run clear.

8. Remove the chicken from the oven and let it rest for 10 to 15 minutes before serving. Enjoy.

Moroccan Chicken and Apricot Tagine

Prepartion time

2 hours 30 minutes

Ingredients

For the Chicken:

- 1 whole chicken (cut into 4 or 8 pieces)
- 3/4 teaspoon salt
- 1 1/4 teaspoons freshly grated ginger
- 1/2 teaspoon saffron threads (crumbled)
- 1/2 teaspoon black pepper
- 1/4 teaspoon white pepper

- 1/4 teaspoon Ras el Hanout, optional
- 1/2 teaspoon turmeric

For the Tagine:

- 3 tablespoons butter
- 2 tablespoons olive oil
- 2 medium onions (grated)
- 3 to 4 cloves garlic (pressed or finely chopped)
- 1 or 2 small pieces of cinnamon stick (about 3 inches)
- Small handful of cilantro sprigs tied into a bouquet
- 1/2 cup chicken broth
- 3/4 cup water

- 3 tablespoons sugar or honey
- 1 cup dried apricots
- 1 teaspoon ground cinnamon
- Handful of fried almonds, optional
- 1 to 2 teaspoons sesame seeds, optional

Instructions

Gather the chicken ingredients.

1. Combine the spices in a bowl large enough to hold the chicken.

2. Add the chicken and toss to evenly coat the pieces with the spices.

3. Gather the remaining tagine ingredients.

4. Over medium-low heat, melt the butter in the base of a large tagine or Dutch oven.

5. Add the olive oil, onions, garlic, and cinnamon stick.

6. Add the seasoned chicken, meat-side down, in a single layer on top of the onions.

7. Place the cilantro bouquet on top. Add the broth to the tagine.

8. In the bowl used to season the chicken, swirl the water to cleanse it of the spices.

9. Add the water to the tagine.

10. Cover and leave the liquids to reach a simmer over medium-low heat.

11. Once simmering, cook the chicken, undisturbed, for 1 hour.

12. Remove 1/2 cup of the cooking liquids and set aside.

13. Carefully turn over the chicken pieces so that they are meat-side up.

14. Cover the pan and continue simmering for another 30 minutes to 1 hour, until the chicken is done and the liquids are thick and reduced.

15. While the chicken is cooking, put the apricots in a small pot and cover with water.

16. Simmer the apricots over medium heat, partially covered, for 10 to 15 minutes, or until tender enough to pinch in half with your fingers.

17. Drain the apricots and return to the pot.

18. Add the sugar (or honey), ground cinnamon, and the 1/2 cup of the reserved cooking liquid.

19. Simmer the apricots gently for 5 to 10 minutes, or until they are sitting in a thick syrup.

20. Discard the cilantro bouquet and cinnamon stick from the tagine.

21. Arrange the chicken on a large serving platter (or simply leave in the base of the tagine). Spoon the apricots and syrup on and around the chicken. If desired, garnish with fried almonds or sesame seeds.

Moroccan Kefta Tagine

Prepartion time

1 hour 50 minutes

Ingredients

For the Tomato Sauce:

- 2 pounds tomatoes (fresh, ripe)
- Optional: 1 medium onion (finely chopped)
- 1/3 cup olive oil
- 3 tablespoons fresh parsley (chopped)
- 3 tablespoons fresh cilantro (chopped)
- 3 to 5 cloves garlic (pressed)
- 1 1/2 teaspoons paprika
- 1 1/2 teaspoons cumin
- 1 1/2 teaspoons salt
- 1/4 teaspoon black pepper
- 1 bay leaf

For the Kefta Meatballs:

- 1 pound ground beef (or lamb, or a combination of the two)
- 1 medium onions (chopped very fine)
- 1 small green pepper (finely chopped)
- 1/4 cup fresh parsley (chopped, plus more for garnish)
- 1/4 cup fresh cilantro (chopped, plus more for garnish)
- 1 to 2 teaspoons paprika
- 1 teaspoon cumin
- 1 teaspoon salt
- 1/2 teaspoon ground cinnamon

- 1/4 teaspoon black pepper
- 1/4 to 1/8 teaspoon cayenne pepper
- Optional: 1 or 2 chili peppers
- 1/4 cup water
- 3 or 4 eggs

Instructions

Prepare the Tomato Sauce

1. Gather the ingredients.

2. Peel, seed, and chop the tomatoes or, if they're very ripe, cut the tomatoes in half, seed them, and grate them.

3. Mix the tomatoes with 1 finely chopped medium onion (if using), olive oil, parsley,

cilantro, garlic, paprika, cumin, salt, black pepper, and bay leaf in the base of a tagine or in a large, deep skillet.

4. Cover and bring to a simmer over medium-low to medium heat. (Note: If using a clay or ceramic tagine on a heat source other than gas, be sure to place a diffuser between the tagine and burner.)

5. Once simmering, reduce the heat a bit and allow the sauce to simmer gently, at least 15 to 20 minutes but longer if you like, before adding the meatballs.

Make the Kefta Meatballs

Gather the ingredients.

1. Combine the ground beef or lamb, onion, green pepper, parsley, cilantro, paprika, cumin, salt, cinnamon, black pepper, and cayenne pepper.

2. Using your hands to knead in the spices and herbs, shape the kefta mixture into very small meatballs the size of large cherries—about 3/4-inch in diameter.

3. Add the meatballs (and chili peppers, if using) to the tomato sauce, along with a little water—1/4 cup is usually sufficient—and cover.

4. Cook for about 30 to 40 minutes, or until the sauce is thick.

5. Add the eggs to the tagine without breaking the yolks.

6. Cover and cook for an additional 7 to 10 minutes, or until the egg whites are solid and the yolks are only partially set.

7. If desired, garnish with fresh parsley or cilantro,and serve immediately. Enjoy!

Moroccan Fish Tagine (Mqualli)

Prepartion time

4 hours 30 minutes

Ingredients

- 2 pounds firm fish or sea eel (whole or in thick slices or steaks)
- 1 batch chermoula marinade
- 2 bell peppers (any color)
- 1/3 cup olive oil
- 1 large onion, cut into rings (optional)
- 1 carrot or celery stalk (cut into thin sticks)
- 2 large potatoes (cut into thin slices)
- 1 teaspoon ginger
- 1 teaspoon salt
- 1/2 teaspoon pepper
- 1/2 teaspoon turmeric
- Pinch saffron threads (crumbled)

- 2 or 3 tomatoes (seeded and cut into thin slices)
- 1 fresh lemon (cut into thin slices) or 1 preserved lemon (quartered)
- A handful of red olives
- Salt and pepper

Instructions

1. Make the Chermoula and Roast the Peppers
2. Gather the ingredients.
3. Make the chermoula marinade. Reserve and refrigerate half of the chermoula, and mix the remaining half with the fish.

4. Cover the fish and refrigerate, allowing it to marinate for two hours or overnight.

5. Roast the peppers, peel and seed them, and cut them into strips. Or, alternatively, slice the raw pepper into rings. Set aside.

6. Pour the olive oil into a tagine, and distribute the onion slices across the bottom. Criss-cross the celery or carrot sticks in the center to form a bed for the fish.

7. Mix the potato slices with the ginger, salt, pepper, turmeric, and saffron, and arrange the potatoes around the perimeter of the tagine. Top the potato with the tomato slices, then distribute the reserved chermoula over the vegetables.

8. Add the fish and its marinade to the center of the tagine, and arrange the strips of pepper on

top of the fish in a decorative manner. Garnish the tagine with the lemon and olives, and sprinkle salt and pepper over all.

9. Cover the tagine and cook over low to medium-low heat for 1 to 1 1/2 hours, or until the fish and potatoes test done. Reduce the sauce if necessary until it is quite thick and mostly oil. (If you feel there is an excessive amount of liquid in the tagine, it's easiest to ladle the sauce into a pan to reduce it, and then pour the sauce back over the fish before serving.)

10. Serve the tagine directly from the dish in which it was cooked, with Moroccan bread for scooping up the fish and sauce.

11. Enjoy!

Moroccan Vegetarian Carrot and Chickpea Tagine

Prepartion time

55 minutes

Ingredients

- 1 large onion (chopped)
- 4 cloves garlic (finely chopped or pressed)
- 3 tablespoons olive oil
- 1 1/4 teaspoons salt, or to taste
- 1 teaspoon ginger
- 1 teaspoon turmeric

- 3/4 teaspoon cinnamon
- 1/2 teaspoon black pepper
- 1/4 teaspoon cayenne pepper
- Optional: 1/8 teaspoon Ras el hanout (or more to taste)
- 2 or 3 tablespoons chopped parsley or cilantro
- 4 or 5 peeled carrots (cut into 1/4-inch thick sticks)
- 1 cup water (half vegetable or chicken broth, if desired)
- 2 to 3 teaspoons honey (or to taste)
- 1 to 2 cups cooked or canned chickpeas (drained)
- Optional: 1 or 2 small chile peppers

- Optional: 1/4 cup golden raisins
- Garnish Optional: Additional parsley or cilantro

Instructions

Gather the ingredients.

1. In the base of a tagine or in a large skillet with a lid, sauté the onions and garlic in the olive oil over medium-low heat for several minutes.

2. Add the salt, ginger, turmeric, cinnamon, black pepper, cayenne pepper, ras el hanout, parsley or cilantro, carrots, and the water.

3. Bring to a simmer over medium-low heat, then continue cooking, covered, until the carrots are nearly cooked to desired tenderness. In a

skillet, this may take up to 25 minutes, in a tagine a bit longer.

4. Stir in the honey and add the chickpeas and optional chile peppers and raisins. Continue simmering until the chickpeas are heated through and the sauce is reduced and thick.

5. Taste, adjust seasoning if desired, and serve garnished with parsley or cilantro.

6. Enjoy!

Moroccan Berber Tagine With Lamb or Beef and Vegetables

Prepartion time

3 hours 55 minutes

Ingredients

- 1 pound beef (or lamb, cut into 2" to 3" pieces)
- 1/4 to 1/3 cup olive oil
- 1 medium onion (sliced)
- 1 medium onion (finely chopped)
- 3 to 4 cloves garlic (finely chopped or pressed)
- 3 to 4 small potatoes (or medium, quartered lengthwise)
- 3 to 4 medium carrots (halved or quartered lengthwise)
- Optional: 4 small zucchini (whole; or may use other veggies)

- 1 small bell pepper (any color, cut into strips or rings)
- 1 small handful parsley (and/or cilantro, tied into a bouquet)
- Optional: 1 small jalapeno or chili pepper
- 1 small preserved lemon (quartered)
- 1 handful olives (green or red/violet)

For the Seasoning:

- 1 teaspoon salt (or to taste)
- 1 teaspoon ginger
- 1/2 teaspoon black pepper
- 1/2 teaspoon turmeric
- 1/2 teaspoon paprika

- 1/2 teaspoon cumin
- Optional: 1/4 teaspoon cayenne pepper
- Optional: 1 pinch saffron threads

Instructions

1. Pour the olive oil into the base of a tagine.

2. Arrange the onion rings across the bottom and scatter the chopped onion and garlic on top.

3. Arrange the meat, bone-side down, in a mound in the center of the tagine. (The taller the mound, the more conical your arrangement of vegetables will be.)

4. Combine the spices in a small bowl.

5. Sprinkle a little less than half of the seasoning over the meat and onions.

6. Place the prepped vegetables in a large bowl.

7. Add the remaining seasoning and toss to coat the vegetables evenly.

8. Arrange the vegetables in a conical shape around the meat.

9. Arrange the bell pepper strips in the center and top with the parsley bouquet and then the jalapeno pepper, Garnish the tagine with the preserved lemon quarters and olives.

10. Add 2 1/2 cups water to the empty bowl and swirl to rinse the residual spices.

11. Add the water to the tagine, cover, and place the tagine over medium coals in a brazier, or

stovetop over medium-low heat. Note that use of a diffuser under the tagine is necessary if using clay or ceramic on an electric stove and recommended for other heat sources as well.

12. Leave the tagine to reach a simmer. This may take a long time, 20 minutes or so; be cautious in feeling the need to increase the heat.

13. Once simmering, continue cooking the tagine over medium-low heat until the meat and vegetables are very tender and the sauce is reduced, up to 3 hours for beef and up to 4 hours for lamb.

14. While the tagine is cooking, you may check the level of the liquids occasionally and add a little water as necessary, but otherwise, try not to disturb the tagine.

15. Do stay alert for the smell of anything burning, and lower the heat if necessary to avoid scorching ingredients and/or cracking the tagine. It is normal, however, for some of the base onions to burn and adhere to the bottom of the tagine as they caramelize and reduce.

16. Remove the cooked tagine from the heat and serve. It will stay warm while covered for 30 minutes.

Moroccan Lamb or Beef Tagine With Peas and Artichokes

Prepartion time

1 hour 30 minutes

Ingredients

- 1 lb. (about 1/2 kg) lamb or beef, cut into 2" to 3" pieces
- 1 medium onion, chopped (plus one more onion, sliced if cooking in a tagine)
- 3 cloves garlic (finely chopped or pressed)
- 2 teaspoons salt
- 2 teaspoons ginger
- 1 teaspoon pepper
- 1 teaspoon turmeric
- 1/4 teaspoon saffron threads (crumbled)
- 2 tablespoons fresh parsley (chopped)
- 2 tablespoons fresh cilantro (chopped)
- 1/2 cup olive oil

- 1 lb. (about 1/2 kg) peas
- 1 lb. (about 1/2 kg) artichoke bottoms
- 1 preserved lemon (optional)

Instructions

1. Pressure Cooker or Conventional Pot Method

2. Combine the meat, onions, garlic, olive oil, parsley, cilantro, and spices (except for the saffron) in a pressure cooker or wide, heavy-bottomed pot. Cook over medium to medium-high heat, uncovered, for about 10 minutes, stirring several times to turn the meat and brown it on all sides.

3. Add about three cups of water, cover, and increase the heat to high until pressure is

achieved or the liquids boil. Reduce the heat to medium and cook with pressure for 25 minutes (or simmer conventionally for 40 to 60 minutes).

4. Add the peas, artichoke bottoms and saffron. If the liquids are not level with the vegetables, add a little more water. Cover, bring back to pressure and cook for 12 to 15 minutes (or simmer for 25 to 30 minutes) until the vegetables are tender. Check the seasoning and If necessary, reduce the liquids until a rich sauce has formed.

5. Serve with Moroccan bread for scooping up the meat and vegetables.

Clay or Ceramic Tagine Method

1. If using freshly shelled peas, parboil them for several minutes; drain, and set aside.

2. Coat the base of your tagine with a little olive oil. Slice an additional onion into rings and distribute the rings on the bottom of the tagine.

3. In a bowl, mix the meat with the remaining olive oil, chopped onion, garlic, spices and chopped cilantro and place over the sliced onions. Add the mixture to the tagine, taking care to arrange the meat in the middle.

4. Surround the meat with the peas, then arrange the artichoke bottoms all around.

5. Swirl about 2 1/2 cups of water in the bowl used for the meat to "rinse" the spices from the side of the bowl, and add this water to the

tagine. Add a little more water if necessary to barely cover the peas.

6. Close the tagine and place over medium-low heat. (A diffuser is necessary if cooking over an electric burner and recommended for other heat sources as well.) Stay patient while the tagine reaches a simmer -- it could take some time. Once the liquids have reached a simmer, continue cooking the tagine for about 3 hours, checking the liquids once or twice in the last hour of cooking and adding a little bit more water only if you feel it's necessary.

7. The tagine is done when you can easily break the meat apart with your fingers. If necessary, continue simmering uncovered to reduce the sauce.

8. Garnish as desired with strips of preserved lemon. Serve the dish directly from the tagine with Moroccan bread on the side for scooping up the meat and veggies.

Moroccan Sausage and Egg Tagine

Prepartion time

40 minutes

Ingredients

- 8 ounces/225 grams merguez (or similar sausage)

- 1 large onion (finely chopped)
- 2 medium tomatoes (peeled, seeded and chopped)
- Handful of olives (green, pitted, sliced)
- 1/2 teaspoon salt
- 1/2 teaspoon cumin
- 1/4 teaspoon black pepper (or 1/8 teaspoon cayenne pepper)
- Small handful of chopped cilantro (or parsley)
- 6 large eggs
- Salt (to taste)
- Cumin (to taste)
- Garnish: cilantro (chopped or parsley)

Instructions

Gather the ingredients.

1. Cook the sausage in a large skillet or in the base of a tagine until the meat tests as done. (If there is a large amount of fat from the sausage, remove the excess, leaving enough to continue cooking. If the sausage was low-fat, you may need to add a little olive oil to the pan at this point.)

2. Add the onion, tomatoes, olives, and seasoning and cook for about 5 minutes.

3. Pour the eggs directly over the sausage and veggies.

4. Break the yolks, and allow the eggs to simmer until set. (To help this along, you can lift the edges of the eggs as they cook and tip the pan

to allow uncooked egg to run underneath and cook faster.)

5. If cooking the eggs in a tagine, cover the eggs and allow them to poach until done.

6. Dust the top of the cooked eggs with cumin and salt to taste, garnish with a little chopped parsley, and serve.

7. Enjoy!

Moroccan Tagine of Shrimp in Tomato Sauce

Prepartion time

1 hour 45 minutes

Ingredients

- 2 pounds 3 ounces/1 kilogram shrimp (large)
- 2 pounds 3 ounces/1 kilogram tomatoes (fresh and ripe)
- 1/3 cup olive oil
- 1 medium onion (finely chopped)
- 7 cloves of garlic (pressed)
- 1 1/2 teaspoon paprika
- 1 1/2 teaspoon cumin
- 1 1/2 teaspoon salt (or to taste)
- 1/2 teaspoon ginger
- 1/2 teaspoon cayenne pepper
- 2 tablespoons fresh parsley (finely chopped)

- 2 tablespoons fresh coriander (finely chopped)
- Optional: 1 bay leaf
- Garnish: parsley (chopped fresh)
- Garnish: black pepper (coarsely ground)
- Garnish: lemon (slices or wedges)

Instructions

Clean the Shrimp

1. Gather the ingredients.
2. Wash the shrimp under running water and drain.
3. Remove the head, legs, and shells (and tails if desired)
4. Devein the shrimp if necessary.

5. Wash the shrimp again and set aside in a colander to drain.

Make the Tomato Sauce

1. Gather the ingredients.

2. Peel, seed, and chop the tomatoes. (Or, if the tomatoes are very soft, you can cut them in in half, seed them and grate them.)

3. Set the tomatoes aside.

4. Place the base of a large tagine over medium-low heat. (The use of a diffuser between the heat source and tagine is recommended.)

5. Add the olive oil and onions and saute gently for several minutes, or until the onions begin to soften.

6. Add the garlic and saute just for a minute or two, until very fragrant.

7. Remember to maintain the low heat, and avoid burning the garlic.

8. Add the tomatoes, spices and herbs and stir to combine.

9. Cover, and allow the tagine to slowly reach a simmer.

10. Do not increase the heat to speed things up.

11. Continue simmering the tomatoes, stirring occasionally, for about 30 minutes, or until the tomatoes can be mashed with the back of a spoon and a thick sauce forms.

Cook the Shrimp

1. Add the cleaned shrimp to the tomato sauce, along with a few tablespoons of water if you feel the sauce should be thinned, and cover.

2. Cook the shrimp for several minutes then stir gently to turn the shrimp over.

3. Continue cooking for several minutes more, until the shrimp are just done.

4. Remove the tagine from the heat.

To Serve

1. When ready to serve, discard the bay leaf and garnish the tagine with chopped parsley, a few turns of the pepper mill and fresh lemon slices. Wedges of lemon may be offered on the side.

2. It is customary to serve the shrimp directly from the tagine, with each person eating from his side of the dish. In lieu of a fork, Moroccan bread is used to scoop up the shrimp and sauce.

3. Enjoy..

Tagine of lamb & merguez sausages

Prepartion time

4 hours 35 minutes

Ingredients

For the chermoula marinade

- 1 tbsp each ground cumin, paprika and turmeric

- 1 tsp hot chilli powder
- 2 large red onions , roughly chopped
- 3 garlic cloves
- thumb-sized piece ginger , roughly chopped
- 200ml/ 7fl oz olive oil
- 200ml/ 7fl oz lemon juice (about 4 lemons)
- 1 tbsp honey
- large handful flat-leaf parsley , roughly chopped
- large handful coriander , roughly chopped

For the tagine

- 6 lamb shanks or a 1kg/2lb 4oz piece lamb or mutton shoulder (if using shoulder ask the butcher to cut it into 10cm chunks on the bone)
- 4 tbsp olive oil
- 2 carrots , sliced
- 2 red onions , sliced
- 12 dried prunes
- 1 tbsp honey
- juice ½ lemon
- 8 merguez sausages (optional)
- 2 preserved lemons , homemade (see recipe below) or bought, pulp scooped out, rinsed and finely sliced
- 2 mint sprigs, to serve

• harissa , to serve (see recipe below)

Instructions

1. For the marinade, roast the spices in a dry pan for a couple mins until fragrant. Put remaining marinade ingredients in a blender and process to a smooth paste, then add the roast spices and blend again to combine. Place the lamb in a large bowl and pour over the marinade. Leave in the paste overnight, or for at least 2 hrs to absorb all the flavours.

2. Heat oven to 160C/140C fan/gas 3. In a large roasting tin, big enough to fit the meat in one single layer, heat the oil and place over a high heat on the hob. Remove the meat from the

marinade, wiping off and reserving any excess, then brown shanks on all sides in the hot oil.

3. Add remaining marinade to the dish along with the carrots, onions and prunes, then pour in 1 litre water. Cover the dish tightly with foil and cook in a low oven for 3½-4 hrs until the meat is tender and falling away from the bone. Add the honey, lemon juice and seasoning and keep warm.

4. If using, fry the sausages until cooked through, then add to the tagine. Serve the meat in a large bowl with the sauce spooned over, then scatter with the preserved lemons and mint, and serve the harissa on the side.

Family meals: Easy lamb tagine

Prepartion time

2 hours 20 minutes

Ingredients

- 2 tbsp olive oil
- 1 onion, finely diced
- 2 carrots, finely diced (about 150g)
- 500g diced leg of lamb
- 2 fat cloves garlic, crushed
- ½ tsp cumin
- ½ tsp ground ginger
- ¼ tsp saffron strands

- 1 tsp ground cinnamon
- 1 tbsp clear honey
- 100g soft dried apricot, quartered
- 1 low-salt vegetable stock cube
- 1 small butternut squash, peeled, seeds removed and cut into 1cm dice
- steamed couscous or rice, to serve
- chopped parsley and toasted pine nuts, to serve (optional)

Instructions

1. Heat the olive oil in a heavy-based pan and add the onion and carrot. Cook for 3- 4 mins until softened.

2. Add the diced lamb and brown all over. Stir in the garlic and all the spices and cook for a few mins more or until the aromas are released.

3. Add the honey and apricots, crumble in the stock cube and pour over roughly 500ml boiling water or enough to cover the meat. Give it a good stir and bring to the boil. Turn down to a simmer, put the lid on and cook for 1 hour.

4. Remove the lid and cook for a further 30 mins, then stir in the squash. Cook for 20 – 30 mins more until the squash is soft and the lamb is tender. Serve alongside rice or couscous and sprinkle with parsley and pine nuts, if using.

Fragrant fish tagine

Prepartion time

1 hour

Ingredients

For the chermoula & fish

- 2 tbsp olive oil
- 4 garlic cloves , roughly chopped
- 4 tsp ground cumin
- 2 tsp paprika
- bunch coriander , chopped
- 1 tsp salt
- juice and zest 1 lemon

- x skinless tilapia fillets
- For the tagine
- 2 tbsp olive oil
- 2 large onions , halved and thinly sliced
- 2 garlic cloves , sliced
- 2 tsp ground cumin
- 2 tsp paprika
- x cans chopped tomatoes
- 500ml fish stock
- 175g pimento-stuffed olive
- 4 green peppers, quartered, deseeded and sliced
- 500g bag baby new potato , halved lengthways

Instructions

1. To make the chermoula, put the oil, garlic, cumin, paprika, three-quarters of the coriander and the salt in a small bowl. Add the lemon juice, then blitz with a hand blender until smooth. Spoon half over the fish fillets and turn them over to coat both sides. Set aside to marinate.

2. Heat the oil and fry the onions and garlic until softened and starting to colour, about 4-5 mins. Add the cumin and paprika and cook for 2 mins more. Add the tomatoes, stock, olives and lemon zest, stir in remaining chermoula and simmer, uncovered for 10 mins.

3. Stir in the peppers and potatoes, cover and simmer for 15 mins until the potatoes are tender. If freezing, reserve half the sauce and chill before freezing.

4. Stir the remaining coriander into the tagine, then arrange the fish fillets on top (if freezing a batch, reserve 4 portions of fish), and cook for 4-6 mins until the fish is just cooked. Serve with basmati rice, boiled with a little saffron if you like.

Lamb, squash & apricot tagine

Prepartion time

1 hour 50 minutes

Ingredients

- 2 tbsp oil
- 1 large onion, finely chopped
- 2 garlic cloves, finely chopped
- 1 tbsp ras-el-hanout
- 1 tsp ground coriander
- 600g lamb leg, diced into 2cm pieces, excess fat trimmed
- 200g butternut squash, diced
- 200g soft dried apricot
- 400g can chopped tomato
- 500ml lamb or beef stock
- zest 1 lemon

- small bunch coriander
- couscous and natural yogurt, to serve

Instructions

1. Heat oven to 200C/180C fan/gas 6. Heat the oil in a flameproof casserole dish, add the onion and cook for 5 mins until softened. Add the garlic and spices and cook for a couple mins more, stirring to prevent them catching and burning.

2. Add the lamb, squash and apricots to the casserole, pour over the tomatoes and stock, season well and bring to the boil. Put the lid on and transfer to the oven. After 1 hr, stir the tagine and return to the oven, uncovered, for a further 30 mins.

3. Check the seasoning. Sprinkle over the zest and coriander, and serve in warm bowls with couscous and yogurt.

North African chicken tagine

Prepartion time

1 hour 40 minutes

Ingredients

- 2 large chicken breasts, skin on

- 4 chicken thighs, bone in and skin on
- 2 tbsp olive oil
- 200g shallots, peeled
- 2 garlic cloves, sliced
- 4cm piece ginger, grated
- 1 tsp cumin seeds, lightly crushed
- 1 tsp coriander seeds, lightly crushed
- 2 small cinnamon sticks
- large pinch saffron threads
- 1 tsp ground ginger
- pinch crushed dried chilli
- 375g peeled butternut squash, cut into chunks
- 500ml chicken stock

- 1 rounded tbsp clear honey
- 2 tbsp roughly chopped coriander

Instructions

1. Heat oven to 180C/160C/gas 4. Cut each chicken breast in half, then season all the chicken. Heat the oil in a mediumsize ovenproof casserole dish. Add the chicken, skin-side down, and brown well all over – you can do it in batches. Remove from the pan and set aside.

2. Lower heat slightly, add the shallots to the pan and cook until golden brown all over. Add the garlic and grated ginger and cook for 30 secs before adding all the spices and cooking for 1 min more.

3. Throw the butternut squash into the pan and stir to coat in the spices. Arrange the chicken, skin side uppermost, on top of the shallots and squash. Pour over the stock and drizzle in the honey. Bring to a gentle simmer, then transfer to the oven to bake for 40 mins until tender. Scatter with the coriander and serve with couscous and a bowl of harissa, if you like.

Pumpkin, cranberry & red onion tagine

Prepartion time

45 minutes

Ingredients

- 3 tbsp olive oil
- 2 red onions , thickly sliced
- 3cm piece fresh root ginger , grated
- 500g/1lb 2oz pumpkin or squash, peeled, deseeded and cut into large chunks
- 1 tsp each cinnamon , coriander, cumin and harissa paste
- 1 tbsp clear honey
- 700g bottle tomato passata
- 50g dried cranberries
- 400g can chickpea , rinsed and drained
- 200g couscous
- 2 tsp vegetable stock granules
- zest and juice 1 lemon

- 3 tbsp toasted flaked almonds
- handful coriander , roughly chopped

Instructions

1. Heat 2 tbsp oil in a pan and fry the onions until lightly coloured. Add ginger, pumpkin and spices, stir, then add honey, passata and cranberries. Bring to the boil.

2. Reduce the heat, cover, then simmer for 20 mins until the pumpkin is tender. After 10 mins, stir in the chickpeas. (If the mixture is a little thick, you can loosen it with some vegetable stock.)

3. Meanwhile, tip the couscous, stock granules and lemon zest into a heatproof bowl. Pour over

300ml boiling water, stir briefly and cover with a plate. Leave for 5 mins. Tip in the lemon juice, almonds and remaining tbsp oil and fluff up with a fork. Scatter the coriander over the tagine and serve with the couscous.

Fruity lamb tagine

Prepartion time

1 hour 45 minutes

Ingredients

- 2 tbsp olive oil
- 500g lean diced lamb
- 1 large onion, roughly chopped

- 2 large carrots, quartered lengthways and cut into chunks
- 2 garlic cloves, finely chopped
- 2 tbsp ras-el-hanout spice mix
- 400g can chopped tomato
- 400g can chickpea, rinsed and drained
- 200g dried apricot
- 600ml chicken stock

To serve

- 120g pack pomegranate seeds
- 2 large handfuls coriander, roughly chopped

Instructions

1. Heat oven to 180C/160C fan/gas 4. Heat the oil in a casserole and brown the lamb on all sides. Scoop the lamb out onto a plate, then add the onion and carrots and cook for 2-3 mins until golden. Add the garlic and cook for 1 min more. Stir in the spices and tomatoes, and season. Tip the lamb back in with the chickpeas and apricots. Pour over the stock, stir and bring to a simmer. Cover the dish and place in the oven for 1 hr.

2. If the lamb is still a little tough, give it 20 mins more until tender. When ready, leave it to rest so it's not piping hot, then serve scattered with pomegranate and herbs, with couscous or rice alongside.

Guinea fowl tagine

Prepartion time

2 hours

Ingredients

- 1 guinea fowl
- a little olive oil
- 2 carrots , cut into chunks
- 2 red onions , cut into chunks
- 6 dried prunes , dates or figs
- rind 1 preserved lemon , cut into strips
- 1 mint sprig, leaves chopped

- harissa to serve

For the chermoula

- 1 large red onion , roughly chopped
- 1 large garlic clove
- 1.5cm piece fresh root ginger , roughly chopped
- 100ml olive oil
- 100ml lemon juice
- ½ tsp Thai fish sauce
- 1 heaped tsp honey
- ½ tsp ground cumin
- ½ tsp ground paprika

- ½ tsp turmeric powder
- ½ tsp hot chilli powder
- 1 handful flat-leaf parsley
- 1 handful coriander

For the couscous

- 200g couscous
- 1 tsp salt
- 100g butter , cubed
- 1 small handful sultanas

Instructions

1. The day before cooking, put all the ingredients for the chermoula in a blender and process until smooth.

2. Pour over the bird and marinate in the fridge overnight.

3. Next day, heat oven to 220C/200C fan/ gas 7. Scrape the chermoula marinade off the bird and set aside.

4. Heat a little olive oil in a large frying pan and brown the bird on all sides over a high heat. Put the carrots, onions, fruit and reserved chermoula into the tagine and place the guinea fowl on top.

5. Pour in about 400ml water – enough to come 1cm from the top of the tagine base.

6. Cover and cook in the oven for about 45 mins, then turn the heat down to 180C/160C fan/gas 4 and cook for another 45 mins.

7. About 15 mins before serving, rinse the couscous in cold water and put in a shallow bowl.

8. Season with salt and scatter with the butter and sultanas.

9. Pour on 200ml boiling water.

10. Cover and leave for 10 mins or until the grains are plump and tender.

11. Open the tagine at the table and stir the preserved lemon and mint into the juices.

12. Serve the couscous and harissa separately.

Lamb tagine with dates & sweet potatoes

Prepartion time

2 hours 30 minutes

Ingredients

- 6 tbsp olive oil
- 4 onions , thinly sliced
- 2 tbsp finely chopped fresh root ginger
- 2kg boneless lamb shoulder, cut into 5cm chunks
- 4 tsp ground cumin
- 2 tsp each paprika and ground coriander
- 2 cinnamon sticks

- 850ml passata
- 700g sweet potato , cut into chunks
- 350g pitted date

To serve

- 100g blanched almond , toasted
- good handful coriander , roughly chopped

Instructions

1. Heat the oil in a large, deep pan.
2. Add the onions, then gently fry until softened, about 5 mins.
3. Stir in the ginger, add the meat in batches, then fry on all sides until lightly coloured.

4. Return all the meat to the pan, stir in the spices and cinnamon sticks, then cook for 1 min.

5. Add the passata and 800ml water, then bring to the boil, stirring. Season well, then cover and simmer for 1½ hrs, until the lamb is tender.

6. Add the sweet potatoes, stir well, cover again, then cook for 20 mins or until the potatoes are just tender.

7. Stir in the dates and heat through for 5 mins. Taste and add more seasoning if necessary.

8. To serve, spoon the tagine into a serving dish and scatter with the almonds and coriander.

Easy chicken tagine

Prepartion time

50 minutes

Ingredients

- 2 tbsp olive oil
- 8 skinless boneless chicken thighs, halved if large
- 1 onion, chopped
- 2 tsp grated fresh root ginger

- pinch saffron or tumeric
- 1 tbsp honey
- 400g carrot, cut into sticks
- small bunch parsley, roughly chopped
- lemon wedges, to serve

Instructions

1. Heat the oil in a large, wide pan with a lid, add the chicken, then fry quickly until lightly coloured.

2. Add the onion and ginger, then fry for a further 2 mins.

3. Add 150ml water, the saffron, honey and carrots, season, then stir well.

4. Bring to the boil, cover tightly, then simmer for 30 mins until the chicken is tender.

5. Uncover and increase the heat for about 5 mins to reduce the sauce a little.

6. Sprinkle with parsley and serve with lemon wedges for squeezing over.

5-a-day tagine

Prepartion time

45 minutes

Ingredients

- 4 carrots, cut into chunks
- 4 small parsnips, or 3 large, cut into chunks

- 3 red onions, cut into wedges
- 2 red peppers, deseeded and cut into chunks
- 2 tbsp olive oil
- 1 tsp each ground cumin, paprika, cinnamon and mild chilli powder
- 400g can chopped tomato
- 2 small handfuls soft dried apricots
- 2 tsp honey

Instructions

1. Heat oven to 200C/fan 180C/gas 6.

2. Scatter the veg over a couple of baking trays, drizzle with half the oil, season, then rub the oil over the veg with your hands to coat.

3. Roast for 30 mins until tender and beginning to brown.

4. Meanwhile, fry the spices in the remaining oil for 1 min – they should sizzle and start to smell aromatic.

5. Tip in the tomatoes, apricots, honey and a can of water.

6. Simmer for 5 mins until the sauce is slightly reduced and the apricots plump, then stir in veg and some seasoning.

7. Serve with couscous or jacket potatoes.

Duck tagine with clementines

Prepartion time

2 hours 30 minutes

Ingredients

- 6 duck legs
- 200g shallot , peeled
- 2 tsp each ground coriander, cumin, ginger and paprika
- 600ml vegetable stock
- 2 tsp clear honey

- juice 1 lemon
- 6 small, firm clementines , peeled
- 3 tbsp chopped coriander
- 2 tbsp toasted sesame seeds

Instructions

1. Heat oven to 190C/fan 170C/gas 5. Put the duck legs in one layer in a large roasting tin or two smaller ones.

2. Sprinkle with salt, then roast for 45 mins.

3. Remove the duck legs to a dish and spoon 3 tbsp of the duck fat into a large, wide pan (reserve the remainder of the duck fat).

4. Add the shallots and fry briefly until just starting to colour.

5. Sprinkle in the spices and mix well.

6. Add the stock, honey, lemon juice, salt and pepper, and bring to the boil.

7. Sit the duck legs on top, cover tightly and cook over a gentle heat for 1-1¼ hrs until the meat is very tender.

8. Meanwhile, heat 1 tbsp of the duck fat in a frying pan, add the clementines and fry all over until glistening and starting to brown.

9. Add to the pan with the duck and cook for a further 15 mins, then sprinkle with coriander and sesame seeds. This dish goes really well with couscous.

Vegetable tagine with chickpeas & raisins

Prepartion time

30 minutes

Ingredients

- 2 tbsp olive oil
- 2 onions , chopped
- ½ tsp each ground cinnamon , coriander and cumin
- 2 large courgettes , cut into chunks
- 2 chopped tomatoes

- 400g can chickpea , rinsed and drained
- 4 tbsp raisin
- 425ml vegetable stock
- 300g frozen pea
- chopped coriander , to serve

Instructions

1. Heat the oil in a pan, then fry the onions for 5 mins until soft.
2. Stir in the spices.
3. Add the courgettes, tomatoes, chickpeas, raisins and stock, then bring to the boil.
4. Cover and simmer for 10 mins.
5. Stir in the peas and cook for 5 mins more.

6. Sprinkle with coriander, to serve.

Vegetable tagine with almond & chickpea couscous

Prepartion time

35 minutes

Ingredients

- 400g pack shallot , peeled and cut in half
- 2 tbsp olive oil
- 1 large butternut squash , about 1.25kg/2 lb 12oz, peeled, deseeded and cut into bite size chunks

- 1 tsp ground cinnamon
- ½ tsp ground ginger
- 450ml strong-flavoured vegetable stock
- 12 small pitted prunes
- 2 tsp clear honey
- 2 red peppers , deseeded and cut into chunks
- 3 tbsp chopped coriander
- 2 tbsp chopped mint , plus extra for spinkling

For the couscous

- 250g couscous
- 1 tbsp harissa (Moroccan chilli paste)
- 400g can chickpea , rinsed and drained

• handful toasted flaked almonds

Instructions

1. Fry the shallots in the oil for 5 mins until they are softening and browned.

2. Add the squash and spices, and stir for 1 min.

3. Pour in the stock, season well, then add the prunes and honey.

4. Cover and simmer for 8 mins.

5. Add the peppers and cook for 8-10 mins until just tender.

6. Stir in the coriander and mint.

7. Pour 400ml boiling water over the couscous in a bowl, then stir in the harissa with ½ tsp salt.

8. Tip in the chickpeas, then cover and leave for 5 mins.

9. Fluff up with a fork and serve with the tagine, flaked almonds and extra mint.

Moroccan tagine

Prepartion time

2 hours 5 minutes

Ingredients

For the chermoula paste

- 2 red onions , chopped
- 3 garlic cloves

- small knob fresh root ginger , peeled
- 100ml/3½ fl oz lemon juice (about 3 lemons)
- 100ml/3½ fl oz olive oil
- 1 tbsp each honey, cumin, paprika, turmeric
- 1 tsp hot chilli powder
- handful coriander , chopped

For the tagine

- 1 tbsp olive oil
- 3 carrots , cut into chunks
- 3 large parsnips , cut into chunks
- 3 red onions , cut into chunks
- 2large potatoes , cut into chunks

- 4 leeks , ends trimmed and cut into chunks
- 12 dried prunes , dates or figs
- 2 sprigs mint , leaves only, finely chopped

Ingredients

1. To make the chermoula, whizz paste ingredients in a blender.

2. Heat oven to 220C/fan 200C/gas 7.

3. Tip the oil and vegetables into a heatproof casserole and cook on the hob until lightly browned, about 7 mins. You may have to do this in two batches.

4. Add the chermoula paste to the casserole, along with the dried fruit.

5. Pour in 400ml water, cover with a lid and cook in the oven for 45 mins.

6. Reduce heat to 180C/fan 160C/gas 4 and cook for another 45 mins.

7. Sprinkle with the mint.

8. Serve on its own or with couscous or crusty bread.

www.ingramcontent.com/pod-product-compliance
Ingram Content Group UK Ltd.
Pitfield, Milton Keynes, MK11 3LW, UK
UKHW022005190726
13853UKWH00004B/1754

9 798520 902911